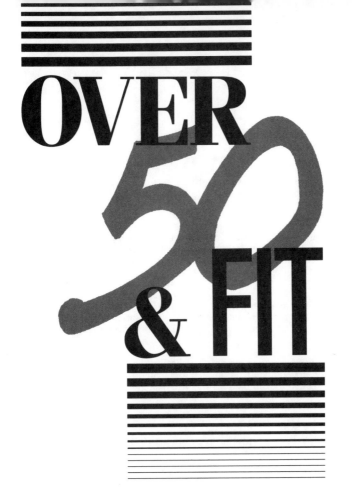

OVER 50 & FIT

Park Nicollet Medical Foundation

CompCare® Publishers

Minneapolis, Minnesota

© 1984 Over 50 and Fit™
Over 50 and Fit is a registered trademark of the Park Nicollet Medical
Foundation, a non-profit organization which was established in 1959
to contribute to the advancement of medical science through research
and education.

This program was developed by Park Nicollet Medical Foundation,
Minneapolis, Minnesota, with a grant from The Medtronic Foundation, a
biomedical engineering company with world headquarters in Minneapolis.

Library of Congress Cataloging-in-Publication Data
Over 50 and fit / Park Nicollet Medical Foundation.
    p. cm.
    Includes index.
    ISBN 0-89638-252-4
1. Exercise for the aged. 2. Exercise. 3. Physical fitness for the
aged. 4. Physical fitness. I. Park Nicollet Medical Foundation. II.
Title: Over fifty and fit.
GV482.6.O94 1991.   91-19116
613.7'0446—dc20   CIP

Cover and interior design by Legend Marketing Communications.

Inquiries, orders, and catalog requests should be addressed to:
CompCare Publishers
2415 Annapolis Lane
Minneapolis, Minnesota 55441
612-559-4800 or toll free 800-328-3330

6	5	4	3	2	1
96	95	94	93	92	91

Our thanks to the Over 50 and Fit™ project staff at Park Nicollet Medical Foundation, Gretchen Porter, R.N., C., M.S., Project Director, Ruth Taylor, B.S.,Debra Terrio, R.N., C., and Ann Chesla, R.N., and to their advisory and consultant personnel, Paul Cederberg, M.D., Park Nicollet Medical Center; William Drake, Deputy General Counsel, Medtronic, Inc.; John B. O'Leary, B.S., M.B., M.D., University of Minnesota; Jane Norstrom, M.A., Exercise Specialist Park Nicollet Medical Foundation; Majlis Parke, Community Representative; Carolyn Peterson, Program Coordinator/ Shape; James Reinertsen, M.D., F.A.C.P., Park Nicollet Medical Center; Robert Spangler, Field Support Manager, Medtronic, Inc.; Charles Stewart, R.P.T., Park Nicollet Medical Center; James Toscano, Vice President, Park Nicollet Medical Foundation.

Special thanks to the staff and participants of senior citizen centers or exercise models who generously assisted in the development of the Over 50 and Fit program.

And to Doug Toft whose editorial expertise has transformed a medically formatted exercise program into a fitness plan for everyone.

Contents

Chapter Three: How to Do the Exercises......27

1

What Fitness Can Do

Just a generation or two ago most people, whatever their age or occupation, got plenty of physical exercise. Often it was only the sick, the very old, and the very rich who were allowed to do much sitting. From sunup to sundown your parents and grandparents kept their bodies moving. They had few machines to do their work for them. They didn't have golf carts, escalators, power lawnmowers, washing machines, or vacuum cleaners. And they didn't have television, that medium of entertainment that has taught a whole generation how to sit without moving for hours at a time.

Modern life is taking its toll. Nowadays our bodies grow old before their time. Muscles turn flabby and soft, and joints stiffen. We get too heavy and tire more easily. It seems the less we move, the less we're able to move.

However, the more we move, the more we want to move. Activity is addictive: it lifts the spirits, energizes the body, and brings a sense of well-being that's hard to beat. Fortunately we don't have to go back to those days of hard physical labor to become more active. We can learn plenty of ways to feel young that are more enjoyable than pushing a plow or scrubbing clothes. This is how participants in the Over 50 and Fit program describe it:

> *My neighbor had to do some persuading to get me to do this program the first time. But now I'm hooked. I'm already beginning to feel stronger, and my grandchildren get a kick out of having a grandmother who wears sweatpants.*

> *I was worried that an exercise program might be too much for this stiff old body of mine. But I discovered that exercise is one of the best prescriptions I've found for pushing back years. I don't want to be any younger, but I sure don't mind feeling younger.*

> *I have a heart condition, so I have to be careful not to overdo it, but I want to be more active. In this program, I go at my own speed. That was probably about a snail's pace at first, but I'm moving faster all the time.*

What Fitness Means

Fitness is a big topic these days. Magazines are featuring articles about it, stores are catering to it, and it seems that everybody is out trying to get fit. Still, some questions go unanswered. For example, what does fitness really mean, and is it only for the young? Listen to these people and decide:

> *I usually work in my yard every morning for about two or three hours before the sun gets too hot. I like every part: gardening, mowing, planting, even weeding. But you know what? The part I think I like best is raking. I feel like I've accomplished something, and besides it's great exercise.*

> *My wife and I take a brisk walk every morning rain or shine. It's a way to get out, breathe the fresh air, see what the weather's like. It just seems like the right way to start the day.*

These people are over 50 and fit. Sure, they're not out running marathons, but fitness means a lot more than jogging for miles on end. Fitness means being able to bend and reach, push and lift. And it means having the stamina to stay active for long periods of time without getting exhausted. These people demonstrate three keys to fitness: strength, stamina, and flexibility. Because they're fit, they're able to stay active and enjoy a full life.

Another Over 50 and Fit participant describes the practical benefits of this view of fitness:

> *I couldn't even touch my toes when we first did stretching exercises, but I worked at them gradually and now I can stretch farther than I could in years. I'm able to reach things way in the back of the cupboard now, and when I bend over to tie my shoes, my body doesn't shout complaints at me. We also do several strengthening exercises, like curl-ups and leg-lifts. All of these strengthening exercises involved either lifting, pushing, or pulling—the same things I do working at home. I've gradually increased my strength so that I can do work that some of my younger friends envy me for. I've got better posture now and fewer aches and pains.*

Aerobic or stamina exercises such as walking and dancing are also an important part of a well-balanced fitness program. During aerobic activities, the large muscles of the body are in constant rhythmic motion. As the muscles work, they need large amounts of oxygen. The lungs and diaphragm work harder to bring the oxygen into the body, and the heart beats faster to pump the oxygen-carrying blood to the muscles. The more demands that are put on the heart, lungs and vessels, the more efficient the whole system becomes. This means a stronger and healthier body for you.

Balancing Exercise

The bodies of highly trained athletes are finely tuned machines. Athletes view their bodies almost as a separate part of themselves. They know that they must care for the body properly, understand how the body runs, and treat it with respect.

Athletes are cautious not to overexert and cause unnecessary damage or injury. When athletes train, they prepare their bodies gradually for the tough workout to come. Before exercising, they take time to warm up muscles, joints, heart, and lungs. When they're finished exercising, they slow down gradually in the same way, cooling down all of the systems that were revved up during the workout.

You may never run a marathon, jump hurdles, or throw a discus, but your body is still a finely tuned machine. Treat it with as much care and respect during exercise as athletes treat theirs. If you warm up and cool down gradually each time you exercise, you won't be as stiff and sore when you're active or afterwards. You'll also be less likely to pull a muscle, get a muscle cramp, or overstress your heart and lungs. When you exercise, include a warm-up period, an aerobic component or a vigorous workout, and a slower cool-down period. Each of these is important to a balanced exercise routine, as this Over 50 and Fit participant points out:

> *Sometimes, when I get to my exercise program, I wonder if I'll ever get my body going. I often feel sluggish and my muscles feel cold and tight. I hardly think my body will ever loosen*

up enough to start moving.
Thank heavens I always begin
slowly and work up to a faster
pace gradually. It usually takes
about ten minutes for my body
to warm up, and then I'm ready
to go.

For optimum results, include three kinds of exercises in your program: those for strengthening, stamina, and flexibility. Stretching exercises are especially designed to make muscles more supple and elastic and increase lubrication to the joints. Both slow movement and stretching are ideal warm-up exercises for getting the body limber and ready for the stamina workout. Stretching exercises are also useful for the cool-down period.

Warm-Up Exercises

When warming up, says another fit person over 50, it pays to be patient:

My body feels pretty rusty when
I first start warming up and
my muscles are all tight like
wound-up rubber bands. I can
barely reach my feet at first,
but I stretch a little and then a
little more and it gets easier
and easier. It's like putting oil
on a rusty hinge.

Warm-up exercises raise the body temperature and help loosen the joints. These exercises also prepare your heart muscle for the stamina workout to come.

Gradually during a 10- or 12-minute warm-up, your

heart rate or pulse begins to increase. Your body literally starts to warm up. By the time you're finished with warm-up exercises, your heart should be ready to do its full load of work in the second phase of the routine, the stamina workout.

Stamina Exercises

As your large muscles move continually and vigorously in aerobic activities, your heart and lungs get a healthy workout as they keep the muscles supplied with oxygen. That's the aim of stamina exercises.

Biking, swimming, jogging, and rowing are all aerobic activities. So are walking and dancing, two activities you can easily adapt to an indoor exercise routine. All of the exercises in the Over 50 and Fit stamina workouts are aerobic.

To make sure you don't overdo it during the stamina workout, you can either keep track of your pulse rate as you exercise or use the Exertion Scale. These methods for monitoring your activity level are explained starting on pages 12 and 13.

Gradual improvement is what counts. Set reasonable goals for yourself each week. When you've achieved them, set new goals. And remember, your only contest is with yourself. Here's how one person described it:

> *I've worked in an office most of my life, which meant a lot of sitting. Since my retirement, arthritis has kept me from getting much exercise. I was really worried that I couldn't do any of the workout exercises and*

believe me, I started very slowly.
Now, I can keep going for much
longer and the walk to the mail-
box—it's a piece of cake.

Cool-Down Exercises

After you've exercised vigorously during the stamina workout, you'll be ready for a gradual cool-down. Have you ever noticed how track runners keep moving, even after they've crossed the finish line? They gradually cool their bodies down. They know that if they don't walk around for a while, their muscles will cramp or get stiff and they may even feel lightheaded.

The cool-down period is just as important for you, if you want to avoid any discomfort after you exercise. For the last 5 or 10 minutes of the exercise routine, gradually ease your pace to allow your pulse to slow down to below 100 beats per minute. And let your muscles cool down and relax.

Getting the Most Out of Your Program

If you want to get the most out of an exercise routine, think of it as only one part of a fitness program. For a total fitness program, exercise three to five times a week. If you're just a once-a-week exerciser, you'll start losing those stamina benefits in two to three days after your exercise session. Exercise every other day or so by doing one or two of the routines explained in this book, taking a walk, or doing some other physical activity that you enjoy.

Once you've made a habit of exercising, you'll find

that the benefits are psychological as well as physical. Studies show that exercise works as a mood lifter and tension reducer. It gives you an overall sense of well-being.

Developing good all-around fitness is a great way to expand your horizons as you age. Instead of doing less as the years go by, you'll be doing more. You'll feel better and be able to enjoy life to its fullest. Remember that you don't stop exercising when you grow older—you grow older when you stop exercising.

About the Program

Over 50 and Fit is one way to have fun getting fit. This program was developed by a panel of physicians, health educators, and other health professionals. They tested the exercises and routines in this book with classes of older adults, finding out what worked for people over age 50. What you're holding in your hand is the result of their teamwork.

After ten weeks of a regular exercise program like Over 50 and Fit, you're likely to have more strength and stamina for your daily activities. Your flexibility will be improved and you'll be able to do more without fear of injury. Your mobility may increase and your self-image will be enhanced. This program is safe, self-paced, and can help to make exercise a regular part of your life.

The rest of this book is divided into four chapters: Exercise Information, How to Do the Exercises, Exercise Routines, and Alternative Exercises. A glossary in the back of this book defines words related to fitness, and the index of exercises can help you locate instructions for a specific exercise quickly.

2

Exercise Information

Self-Monitoring

You are different from anyone else. You're unique in age, in how active you've been, and in your own physical condition. It's these differences that determine how much you can take on when you begin exercising. To exercise safely, begin at the pace that suits you. It doesn't matter that others can touch their toes, and you can't, or that someone can do more leg lifts than you can. To get the most out of an exercise program, view it as achieving a personal goal, not as a contest with others. Listen to your body. If it says slow down and don't push so hard, obey it.

Over 50 and Fit is designed to provide a safe, effective, and enjoyable fitness program tailored to individual needs. Every person reacts differently to physical activity, so it is important that you monitor your own response to the exercise program. Two methods you can use to judge whether you are pacing yourself safely are 1) taking your pulse and 2) checking the Exertion Scale.

How to Take Your Pulse

Here is an easy way to take your pulse. You will need a watch or clock that measures seconds.

1. **Rest two fingers of your watch hand on the thumb knuckle of your other hand.**

2. **Slide the fingers down the thumb toward your wrist until you feel the wrist bone.**

3. **Feel your pulse on the palm of your wrist, approximately a quarter-inch from your wrist bone.**

4. **Now, with your fingers resting gently over the pulse, count the number of beats you feel for six seconds.**

5. **Add a zero to this number to get your one-minute heart rate. For example, if you count seven beats, your pulse is 70.**

Scientists have identified a safe pulse range, called the Target Heart Rate Zone, which is adjusted for age. If you keep your pulse within that range, you are exercising safely yet strenuously enough to benefit from the exercise.

Find your age on the chart on page 13. Then follow across to the numbers in the middle column to find your Target Heart Rate Zone for the six-second count, and follow over to the last column to find your Target Heart Rate Zone for the one-minute count. For example, if you are 60 years old, your Target Heart Rate Zone will be 96 to 128 heartbeats per minute.

Target Heart Rate Zone

Age	Pulse Rate 6 sec.	1 min.	Age	Pulse Rate 6 sec.	1 min.	Age	Pulse Rate 6 sec.	1 min.
50	10-13	101-136	60	10-13	96-128	70	9-12	90-120
51	10-13	100-135	61	9-13	95-127	71	9-12	89-119
52	10-13	100-134	62	9-13	95-126	72	9-12	88-118
53	10-13	100-134	63	9-13	94-126	73	9-12	88-118
54	10-13	99-133	64	9-12	94-125	74	9-12	87-117
55	10-13	99-132	65	9-12	93-124	75	9-12	87-116
56	10-13	98-131	66	9-12	92-123	76	9-11	86-115
57	10-13	98-130	67	9-12	92-122	77	9-11	86-114
58	10-13	97-130	68	9-12	91-122	78	8-11	85-114
59	10-13	96-129	69	9-12	90-121	79	8-11	85-113
						80	8-11	84-112
						Over	8-11	84-112

The length of time you should exercise vigorously during the stamina workout will be determined by how active you are. If you've been a daily walker, for example, you may be able to keep your heart in the target zone for 15 to 25 minutes right from the beginning. On the other hand, if you lead a more sedentary life, you may need to begin by exercising for only a few minutes and then build up to a goal of sustained activity for 25 minutes.

If you're over 50 and have been inactive for a while, start by exercising for five minutes in the target zone the first week. Once you feel comfortable with that, try eight minutes and keep progressing gradually each week. Your goal should be about 15 to 25 minutes of exercising in your target zone. But don't worry if you don't quite reach that mark.

Exertion Scale

The second method for estimating how hard you are exercising is called the Exertion Scale. It's especially useful for people who are taking certain blood pressure medicines that keep their pulse low.

By listening to your own body—how heavily you are breathing and how tired you feel—you can get a good indication of how hard your heart is working. Your own estimation of how hard you are exercising is surprisingly accurate compared to your actual pulse rate.

Exertion Scale:

1. Extremely light

2. Very light

3. Light but noticeable

4. Moderate

5. Somewhat hard

6. Hard

7. Very hard, breathing heavy

Rate yourself on the Exertion Scale for your own level of exertion. Compare your breathing and heart-beat from the time you begin to exercise until you finish. Aim to exercise at an exertion level of four to six. Reaching seven on the scale indicates that you should slow down a little.

Remember, effective exercise is self-paced and self-monitored. Don't rely on anyone to tell you when to stop exercising. Keep in mind that you are not in competition with anyone else, and don't push yourself too hard.

The following words from an Over 50 and Fit participant describe how to use the Exertion Scale:

> *When I start exercising, I don't feel tired at all, probably a level of one or two on the exertion scale. As I exercise more vigorously, my heart starts beating a little harder and I'm probably up to a level of three or four on the scale. When I'm really pushing myself and breathing hard, I'm at a level of six. At this rate my heart is beating fast and I feel pretty tired. My body tells me that it's time to slow down.*

A handy guideline to remember is this: If you can talk while you're exercising, you're probably within a safe limit. If you notice any of the warning signs listed below while exercising, see your doctor before continuing with the program.

When you become a regular exerciser, you probably won't need to continue taking your pulse or using the Exertion Scale at regular intervals. The more you exercise, the more you understand your body and its limits. You'll monitor your efforts almost unconsciously and have fun.

Caution Signs to Stop Exercising

Aerobic exercises are safe if you begin gradually and stay within your own limits. It's normal for your heart to pound and your breathing to become faster, and you may also perspire as you exert yourself. But if any of the following warning signs appear, stop exercising until you've revised your program or consulted with your physician:

▶ Unusual heart action, such as fluttering or sudden slow pulse

▶ Pain or pressure in your chest, arm, or jaw

▶ Dizziness, lightheadedness, or nausea

▶ Cold sweat or pallor

▶ Extreme breathlessness

▶ Rapid heartbeat for 5 or 10 minutes after you stop exercising

▶ Prolonged fatigue even 24 hours later

▶ Flare-up of arthritis or painful joints

▶ Steady joint pain lasting more than two hours

Pacing: Warm-Ups, Aerobics, and Cool-Downs

To get the most from exercise, it's important to pace yourself throughout your workout. As mentioned in Chapter One, Over 50 and Fit exercise sessions are structured to let you prepare your muscles for more vigorous activity with three kinds of exercise: slow warm-up routines, aerobic routines, and relaxing cool-down routines.

When you begin the Over 50 and Fit program, start with 10 to 12 minutes of warm-up routines made up of stretching exercises. As you do these exercises, your heart rate or pulse gradually begins to increase and your body literally starts to warm up. By the time you're finished with the warm-up routines, your heart should be ready to do its full load of work.

Again, a sensible plan for aerobic exercise is to start exercising vigorously enough to raise and maintain your heart rate in your Target Heart Rate Zone for five minutes. If that is a comfortable pace, gradually work up to maintaining your heart rate in your Target Heart Rate Zone (exercising at a level of 5 or 6 on the Exertion Scale) for 15 to 25 minutes.

The length of time you can exercise vigorously during the aerobic workout will be determined by how active you are. If you're a daily walker, for example, you may be able to keep your heart rate in your Target Heart Rate Zone for 15 to 25 minutes right from the beginning.

To increase your stamina—that is, to strengthen the heart and lungs—do aerobic exercises three to five times per week. You will start to lose the stamina benefits after about two days with no exercise, so do aerobic exercises regularly.

Taking time to cool down after aerobic exercise is important in an exercise program. During the 5- to 10-minute cool-down routines, you will decrease your pace and allow your pulse to return to less than 100 beats per minute.

Exercise Tips

Exercise and Breathing

Proper breathing makes a big difference in an exercise program. Many of us have the habit of holding our breath while we exercise, which puts stress on the cardiovascular system. Keeping your oxygen level high allows you to exercise more easily and receive maximum benefits. Taking a few slow, deep breaths before you begin each exercise will help bring the needed oxygen into your system.

Useful guidelines for breathing include the following:

▶ Breathe in when the exercise expands your rib cage, and breathe out when the exercise contracts your rib cage.

▶ Breathe in when your arms and legs are stretched away from the body, and breathe out when your arms and legs are close to the body.

▶ Do some slow, deep breaths at the end of your exercise routine to help you relax and reduce your heart rate.

▶ Breathe in during the relaxation phase of an exercise and breathe out during exertion.

Exercise and Eating

Avoid exercising on a full stomach. Vigorous exercise interferes with the digestive process for at least one hour before or after a meal. However, be sure to eat a well-balanced diet, because you will burn more calories with regular exercise.

Exercise and Alcohol

Exercise and alcohol don't mix. To get the most out of your fitness program, don't drink for at least four hours before exercising. Alcohol interferes with oxygen transfer to the muscles and constricts the blood vessels in the heart.

Exercise and Water

Drink enough water to quench your thirst. You lose a lot of body fluid when you exercise heavily or in warm weather. Loss of body fluid reduces the body's ability to get adequate circulation to working muscles and inhibits the body's ability to cool itself through perspiration. Water replenishes the body better than other fluids because it is easily absorbed into your system.

Exercise and the Weather

Don't exercise in extreme temperatures! It puts an added strain on your heart and blood vessels. In cold weather, dress properly and warm up your muscles before starting to exercise. In warm weather, wear cool, absorbent clothes and slow down your pace. Cool down when you're finished exercising until your pulse rate is below 100 beats per minute.

What to Wear

Comfort is the key. Loose-fitting clothes allow you to move freely. Clothing with some cotton content is good for absorption. A long- or short-sleeve knit top and knit slacks that stretch are good examples of what to wear. Shoes should be flexible and well fitting. Tennis shoes or low-heeled oxfords are good choices. Stockings should be fresh and absorbent.

Injuries and Illness

The best way to avoid injury is to exercise within your limitations. If you strain yourself during exercise, apply ice to muscles and joint injuries for the first 24 hours to minimize swelling. Postpone or cut back on exercise if you have a cold or temporary illness. Take time to recuperate before resuming your exercise program.

Exercise and Wheelchairs

Many of the exercises in the Over 50 and Fit program can be done by people in wheelchairs. Modify the routines by substituting movements with your legs, feet, upper body, or arms for other movements you find difficult. If one limb has less strength, use the stronger limb to help it through the motion. Go through the movements slowly, and be sure your wheelchair is locked and stable.

Showers, Whirlpools, and Saunas

Cool off after aerobic exercise with a slow walk or cool-down routine. Hot showers, whirlpools, and saunas should be avoided after strenuous exercise because they tend to speed up your heart rate.

Exercises to Avoid

Exercises that put your muscles and joints into extreme or rapid motion can cause injury. Avoid the following exercises.

Double Leg Lift

Lifting legs together while lying on your back puts stress on lower back muscles.

Double Straight Leg Circles (sitting in chair)

Extending both legs and rotating them straight from a sitting position puts stress on the lower back muscles.

Straight Leg Sit-ups

Doing sit-ups with legs straight puts added stress on lower back muscles.

Swan Stretch

Stretching up with feet and hands while lying on your stomach puts stress on the spine.

Deep Knee Bends

Alternating quickly between a standing position and a squat pinches the knee joint.

Isometric Exercises

These exercises involve contracting muscles without moving your arms or legs. Doing so may lead you to hold your breath, which can increase your blood pressure and lead to dizziness and fainting.

Head Tilt

Tilting the head backward puts stress on the spine and can cause dizziness and neck spasms.

Toe Touches

Touching the toes with straight knees puts added stress on the lower back.

Bouncing or Jumping Jacks

Any kind of bouncing or jumping exercise puts stress on the leg joints, unless it is done on a soft, resilient surface such as a jogging trampoline.

Exercise and Weight Control

Over 50 and Fit is not primarily a weight-loss program, but you may lose weight and firm up with this program.

Body weight is the result of energy balance. If the calories you consume equal the number of calories you burn, your weight will remain the same. You gain weight by consuming more calories than you're burning. If you burn more calories through increased activity and keep your calorie intake constant, you'll lose weight. For example, a 15- to 20-minute daily walk will burn off about 15 pounds a year.

It's important to remember that the calories you consume should contain the nutrients your body needs. A balanced diet includes foods from the four major food groups: meat, fish and poultry; fruits and vegetables; breads and cereals; and dairy products. If you are interested in learning more about weight control, ask your physician or community nutritionist.

The following list of activities shows the amount of calories burned per hour. All amounts are approximate because exact calories burned depends on body weight and activity intensity.

Very Light (50 – 149 cal.)

Typing
Standing
Cooking
Reading
Writing

Sitting
Knitting
Dusting
Sewing
Ironing

Moderate (150 – 299 cal.)

Walking: 2-3 MPH
Housework: windows,
  vacuuming, mopping
Light gardening: hoeing,
  raking

Planting
Office filing
Driving a car
Carpentry

Vigorous (300 – 449 cal.)

Walking: 4 MPH
Scrubbing floors
Biking
Heavy gardening:
  weeding, shoveling

Mowing lawn
Carrying
  groceries
Dancing

Strenuous (450 cal. and over)

Jogging
Running
Walking up hills
Sawing
Chopping wood

Shoveling
  snow
Cross-country
  skiing
Tennis
Swimming

Making Exercise a Lifestyle

Fitness is a lot more than lifting weights or jogging for miles. Fitness means being able to bend, push, and lift. It means having the stamina to stay active for long periods of time without getting exhausted.

A balanced exercise program includes exercises for strength, stamina, and flexibility. Daily activities such as working in the garden or a brisk walk are great because they help to improve your strength, stamina, and flexibility all at the same time. Unfortunately, most people don't get a consistent exercise balance without the benefit of a regular fitness program.

Over 50 and Fit is a good supplement to daily activities because it provides a ready-made balance of what your body needs to stay in shape. This program teaches the basic principles of balanced fitness so you can incorporate exercise into your daily activities.

3

How to Do the Exercises

The exercises in this chapter are presented in recommended order. Once you have learned the individual exercises, then combine them into routines as explained in Chapter Four. To make sure you do the movements correctly, review the exercise instructions from time to time.

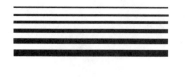

Neck Pendulum

Stretches neck and upper back

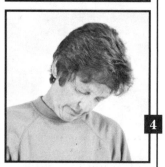

Start standing erect with arms relaxed.

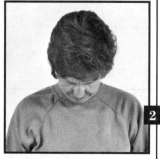

Slowly lower head.

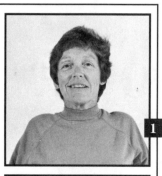

Roll head to one side.

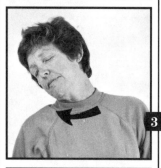

Slowly roll head to other side and return.

Tip: Try not to drop your head back past your shoulders.

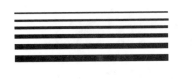

Head Turn

Stretches neck muscles

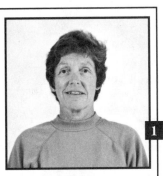

1 Start standing erect, looking straight ahead.

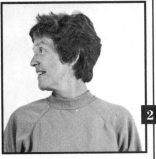

2 Look toward one shoulder.

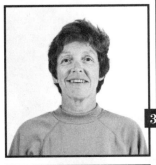

3 Look straight ahead.

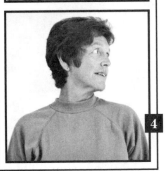

4 Look toward other shoulder and return to starting position.

Tip: Don't let your chin drop.

Shoulder Circles

Stretches shoulder muscles and releases upper back tension

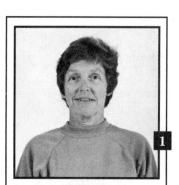

Start standing erect with shoulders relaxed.

Circle shoulders backward.

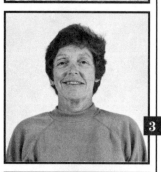

Return to starting position.

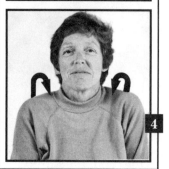

Circle shoulders forward and return to starting position.

Tip: This exercise is best done relaxed. Don't clench fists.

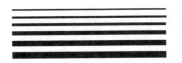

Shoulder Shrugs

Strengthens and relaxes shoulder muscles

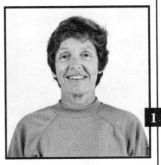

Start standing erect with shoulders relaxed.

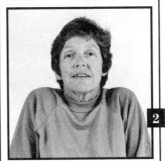

Raise shoulders and then relax.

Single Arm Circles

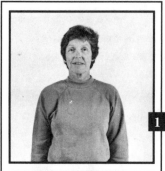

Start standing erect with arms relaxed.

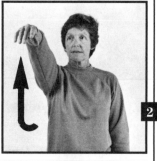

Circle one arm forward, up and around.

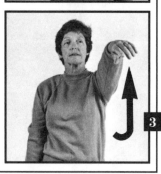

Circle other arm forward, up and around.

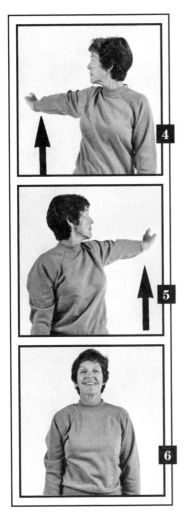

Circle first arm backward, up and around.

Circle other arm backward, up and around.

Return to starting position.

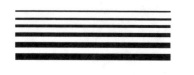

Overhead Arm Reach

Stretches upper arm and back

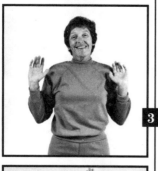

1 Start standing erect with hands in front of shoulders and palms out.

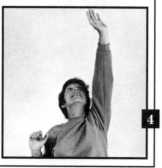

2 Reach up with one arm.

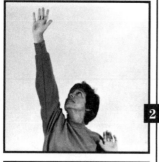

3 Return to starting position.

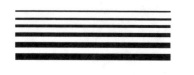

4 Reach up with other arm and return to starting position.

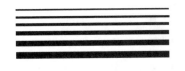

Forward Reach

Stretches upper back

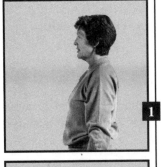

Start standing erect with arms relaxed.

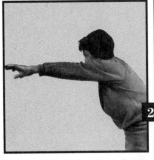

Reach forward with both arms.

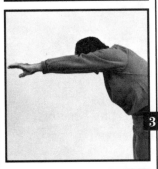

Lower head and stretch forward.

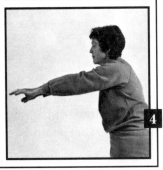

Raise head and return to starting position.

Tip: Try not to bend at waist.

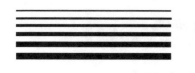

Side Stretch

Stretches trunk muscles

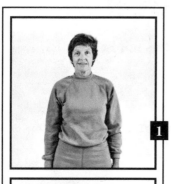

1 Start standing with legs shoulder-width apart, and arms relaxed.

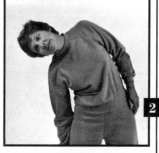

2 Slide one arm down side of leg.

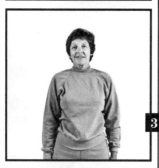

3 Return to starting position.

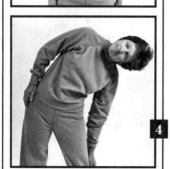

4 Slide other arm down side of leg and return to starting position.

Tip: Try not to lean forward or backward.

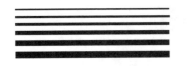

Side Lunge

Stretches inner thigh muscles

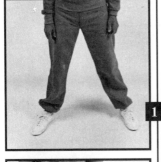

1 Start standing with legs apart and arms relaxed.

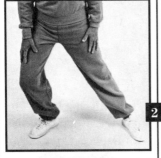

2 Bend one knee and shift weight to that side.

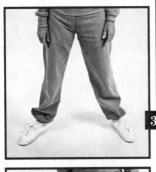

3 Return to starting position.

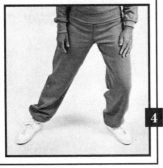

4 Bend other knee and shift weight to that side.

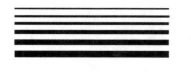

Calf
Stretch

Stretches calf muscles

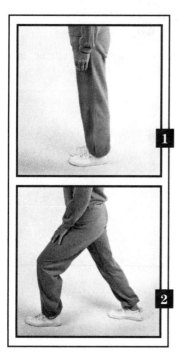

1 Start standing with feet together and arms relaxed.

2 Step forward with one leg, bending the knee. Keep back leg straight with heel on floor.

3 Relax and repeat with other leg.

Tip: People with balance problems may need the support of a chair or wall.

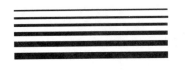

Forward Stretch

Stretches inner thigh and lower back muscles

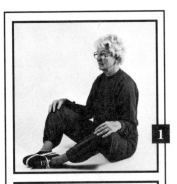

Start sitting on floor, bottoms of feet together or ankles crossed, and hands on knees.

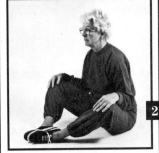

Slowly lean forward.

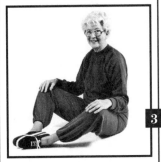

Slowly return to starting position.

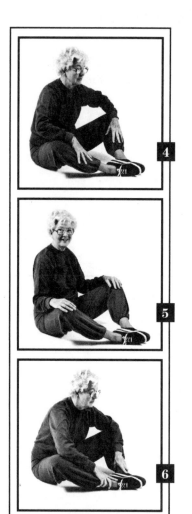

4 Place hands on shins and lean forward.

5 Return to starting position.

6 Place hands on ankles and slowly lean forward. Return to starting position.

Tips: Move slowly, don't force stretch. People with total hip replacements should omit this exercise.

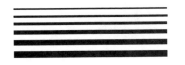

Straddle Stretch

Stretches back of legs and lower back

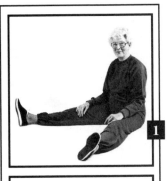

Start sitting on floor with legs apart.

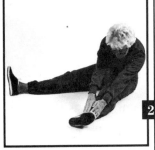

Without bending knees, reach toward one foot with both hands.

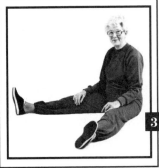

Return to starting position.

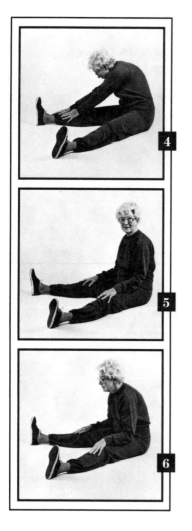

Without bending knees, reach toward other foot with both hands.

Return to starting position.

Lean forward with hands on both legs. Return to starting position.

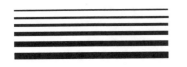

Flexed Straddle Stretch

Stretches calf muscles

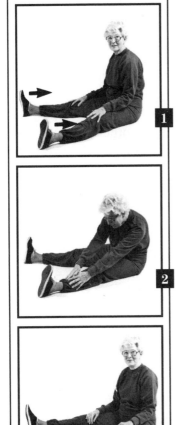

1 Start sitting on floor, with legs apart and toes flexed.

2 Without bending knees, reach toward one foot with both hands.

3 Return to starting position.

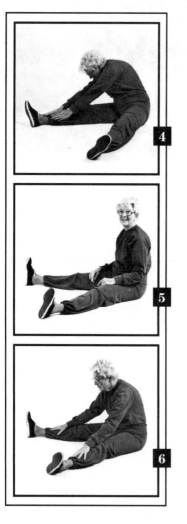

Without bending knees, reach toward other foot with both hands.

Return to starting position.

Without bending knees, place one hand on each leg, and lean forward. Return to starting position.

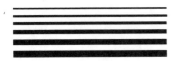

Combination Stretch

Stretches legs, upper back, and hips

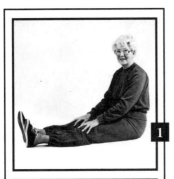

Start sitting on floor with legs together.

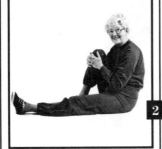

Bring one knee up to chest.

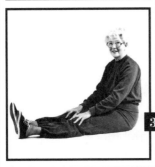

Straighten leg.

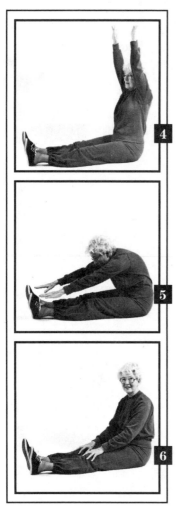

4 Stretch both arms over head.

5 Reach toward toes.

6 Return to starting position and repeat with other leg.

Tip: People with total hip replacement should omit step 2 for the affected side.

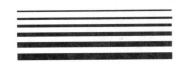

Elbow Circles/ Elbow Press

Loosens shoulder joints, upper back, and arms

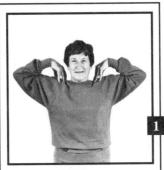

1 Start walking slowly with hands on shoulders.

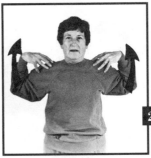

2 Circle elbows backward.

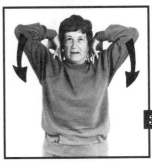

3 Circle elbows forward.

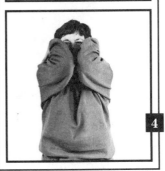

4 Touch elbows together in front and return to starting position.

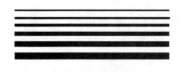

Walks

Stretches feet and legs

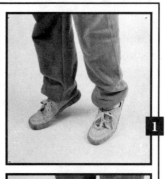

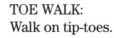

TOE WALK:
Walk on tip-toes.

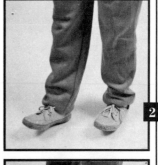

HEEL WALK:
Walk on heels.

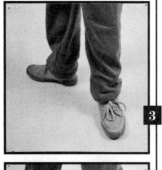

DUCK WALK:
Walk with toes pointed out.

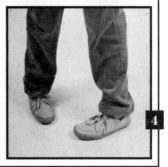

PIGEON WALK
Walk with toes pointed in.

Tip: People with total hip replacement should omit DUCK WALK and PIGEON WALK.

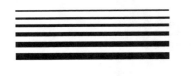

Lower Leg Lift

Strengthens thighs and abdomen

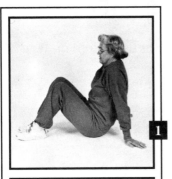

1 Start sitting on floor with knees bent, supporting weight with arms.

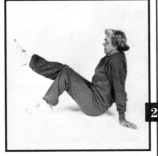

2 Lift one leg at knee.

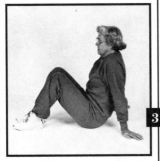

3 Return to starting position.

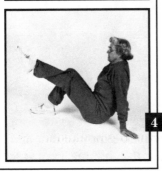

4 Lift other leg at knee and return to starting position.

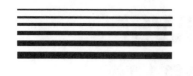

Total Leg Lift

Strengthens abdomen, legs, and back

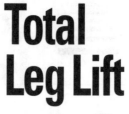

Start sitting on floor, knees bent. **1**

Bring one knee to chest. **2**

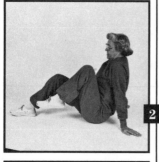

Straighten leg, pointing toe toward ceiling. **3**

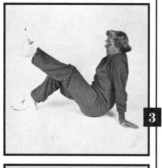

Lower straightened leg to floor. Return to starting position and repeat with other leg. **4**

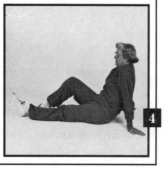

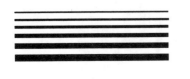

Curl Down

Strengthens abdomen

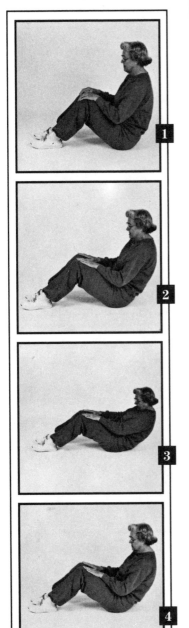

1 Start sitting on floor, with hands on bent knees.

2 Curve your back.

3 Lower yourself halfway to the floor.

4 Return to starting position.

Tips: Back is kept rounded, not arched. Breathe regularly, don't hold your breath.

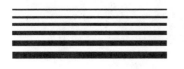

Curl Up

Alternative to curl down

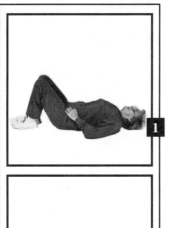

Start lying down with knees bent and feet on floor.

Raise head off floor, chin toward chest, reaching toward knees with both hands.

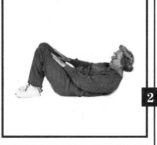

Roll shoulders off floor as you touch knees.

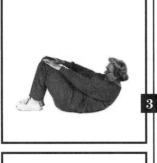

Roll shoulders back down and relax.

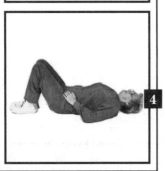

Tips: Be sure head comes up first. Try not to arch back. Don't hold breath. Take slow, even breaths.

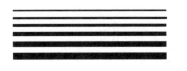

Knee Drop

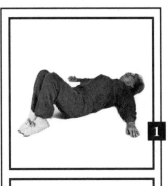

**Stretches abdomen
and side muscles**

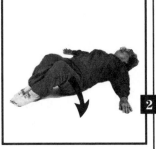

1 Start lying down with knees bent
and arms extended on either side
of your body.

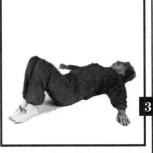

2 Lower knees to one side keeping
both shoulders flat on the floor.

3 Return to starting position.

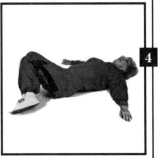

4 Lower knees to other side,
keeping shoulders flat on the
floor. Return to starting position.

Tips: Watch to make sure shoulders
are flat on the floor. Keep the movement gentle to avoid lower back
injury. People with total hip replacement should omit this exercise.

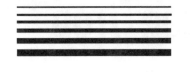

Leg Lowering I

Strengthens abdomen and legs

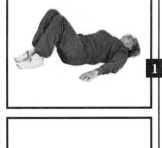

Start lying down with knees bent, feet on the floor, knees and arms extended on either side of your body.

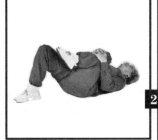

Bring one knee toward chest.

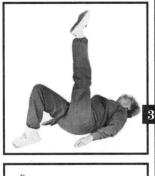

Straighten leg, pointing toe toward ceiling.

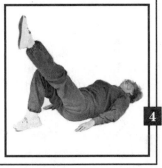

Lower straightened leg to floor. Return to starting position and repeat with other leg.

Tip: People with total hip replacement should omit this exercise.

Leg Lowering II

Strengthens abdomen and legs

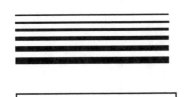

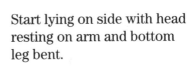
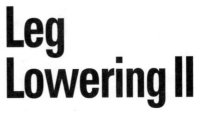

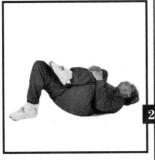

Start lying on side with head resting on arm and bottom leg bent.

Without bending knee, raise leg toward ceiling.

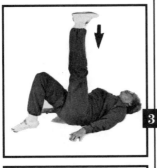

Straighten leg, toes flexed.

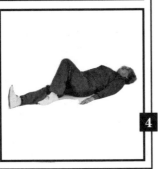

Lower straightened leg to floor. Return to starting position and repeat with other leg.

Tip: People with total hip replacement should omit this exercise.

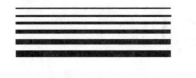

Side Leg Lift

Strengthens outer thigh

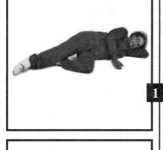

1 Start lying on side with head resting on arm and lower leg bent.

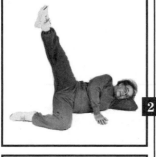

2 Raise top leg toward ceiling, keeping knee straight.

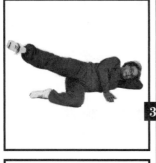

3 Lower leg to floor.

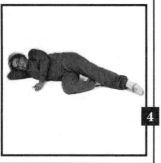

4 Turn over on other side in the same starting position and repeat.

Tips: Lift leg straight toward ceiling. Don't bend at knee. People with total hip replacement should omit this exercise.

Pelvic Tilt

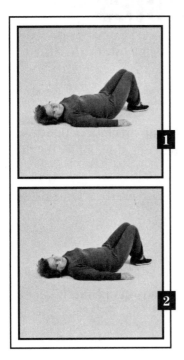

1 Start lying on back with knees bent.

2 Tighten stomach muscles, flatten the small of the back down against the floor, hold, and then relax.

Wrist Circles

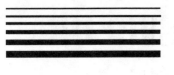

Keeps wrist joints flexible

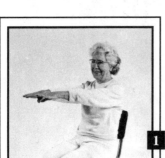

1 Start sitting on chair with arms stretched out at shoulder height.

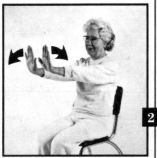

2 Circle hands in one direction.

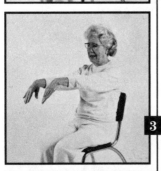

3 Circle hands in other direction.

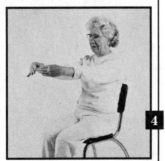

4 Relax.

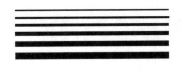

Palm Rotation

Maintains shoulder flexibility

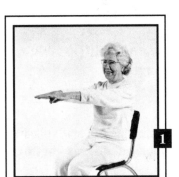

Starting sitting in chair with arms stretched out at shoulder height.

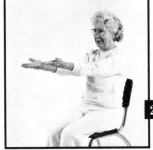

Rotate palms up.

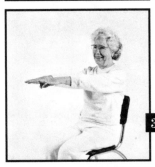

Rotate palms down.

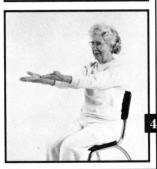

Rotate palms up and relax.

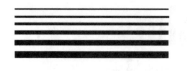

Finger Flex

**Maintains flexibility
and strength**

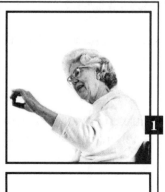

Start sitting on chair with elbow
bent. Touch thumb and forefinger.

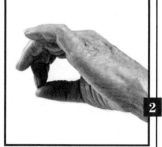

Touch thumb and middle finger.

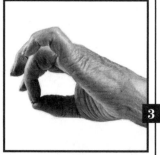

Touch thumb and ring finger.

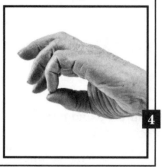

Touch thumb and little finger. Do
in reverse order and repeat with
other hand.

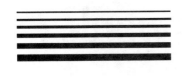

Lower Leg Lift

Strengthens abdomen and thighs

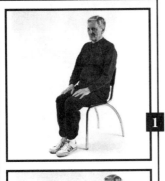

1 Start sitting in chair with hands on knees.

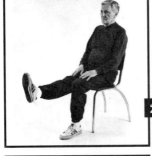

2 Lift one leg at knee.

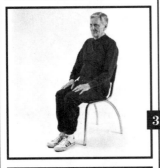

3 Return to starting position.

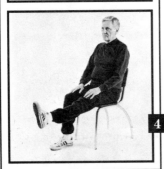

4 Lift other leg at knee and return to starting position.

Tip: Keep lower back against chair.

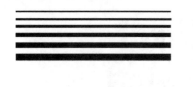

Forward Stretch

Stretches back and hips

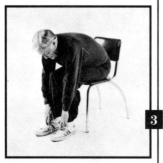

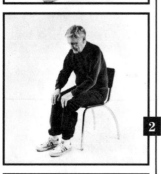

1. Start sitting in chair with hands resting on knees.

2. Bend forward slowly. Start with lowering chin to the chest, then gradually curl down toward the floor.

3. Reach down toward your feet.

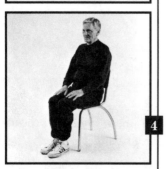

4. Return to starting position.

Tip: Watch out for balance problems.

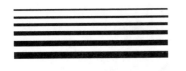

Crossed Ankle Lift

Strengthens legs and stomach

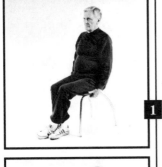

1 Start sitting in chair with ankles crossed holding sides of chair.

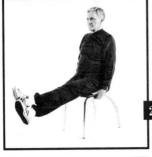

2 Lift lower leg supporting weight of upper leg.

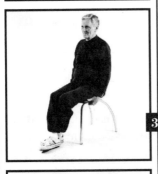

3 Return to starting position. Cross ankles opposite way.

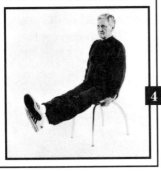

4 Lift lower leg supporting weight of upper leg and return to starting position.

Tips: Breathe normally. Stabilize yourself by holding sides of chair.

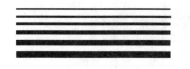

Ankle Circles

Keeps ankle joints loose

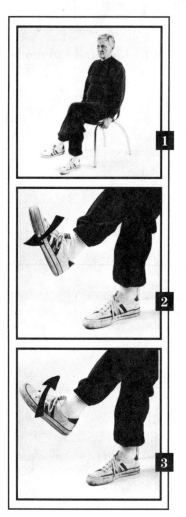

1 Start sitting in chair with legs crossed at knee.

2 Circle upper foot clockwise.

3 Circle same foot in reverse direction. Repeat with other foot.

Tips: People with total hip replacement should not cross legs while doing this exercise.

Body Twist

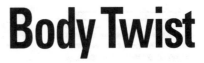

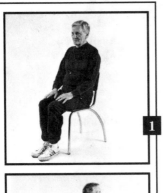

Strengthens trunk muscles

1 Start by sitting on chair with back straight, hands in lap.

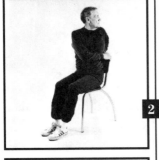

2 Twist to one side grasping back of chair.

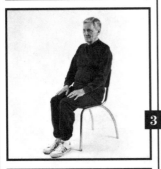

3 Return to starting position.

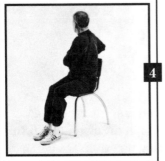

4 Twist to other side grasping back of chair and return to starting position.

Tips: Exercise should be done gently. Do not do this exercise if you have had back surgery.

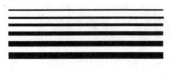

Total Leg Lift

**Strengthens abdomen
and lower back**

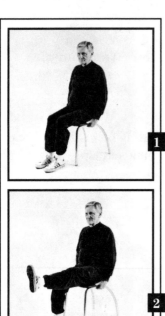

1 Start sitting, holding sides
of chair.

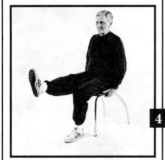

2 Straighten and lift one leg, raising
thigh off chair.

3 Return to starting position.

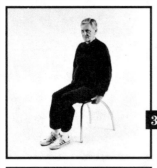

4 Straighten and lift other leg,
raising thigh off chair, and return
to starting position.

Tip: Keep back pressed against
chair. Do not arch back.

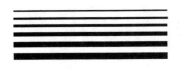

Heel Lifts
with Half Knee Bends

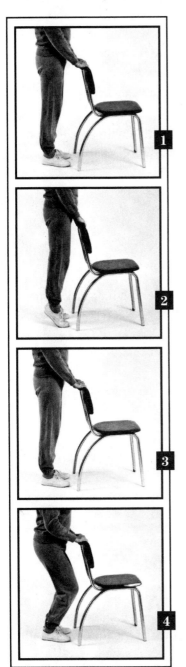

1 Start standing behind chair, holding on to back of chair.

2 Raise up on toes.

3 Bring heels back to the floor.

4 Keeping heels on floor, do half knee bend and come back up.

Tip: Keep back straight throughout exercise.

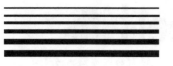

Leg Swings

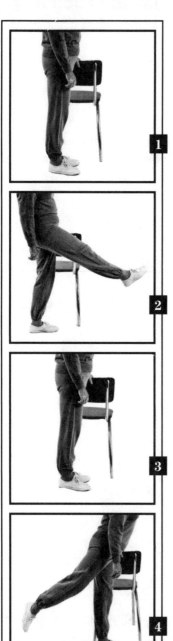

Strengthens upper legs and buttocks

1 Start standing with side to chair, holding on to back of chair.

2 Swing outer leg forward from hip.

3 Return to starting position.

4 Swing outer leg back from hip and return. Repeat on other side.

Tip: Try not to kick too high; swing easy.

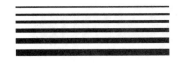

Forward Lunge

Stretches calf muscles

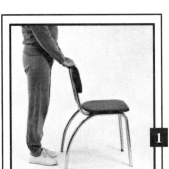

1 Start standing away from chair, holding on to back of chair.

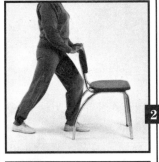

2 Step forward with one leg, keeping front knee bent and back heel on floor.

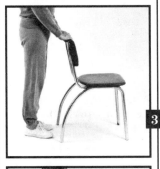

3 Return to starting position.

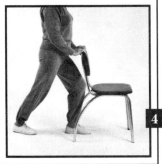

4 Step forward with other leg, keeping front knee bent and back heel on floor; return to starting position.

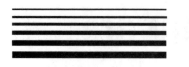

Side Lunge

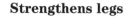

Strengthens legs

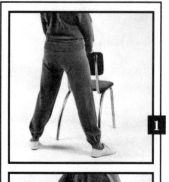

1 Start standing at back of chair with legs apart, holding on to back of chair.

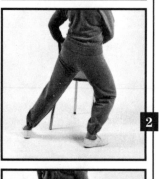

2 Bend one knee and shift weight to that side.

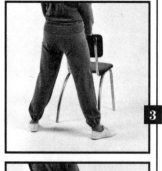

3 Return to starting position.

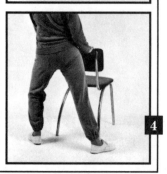

4 Bend other knee and shift weight to that side; return to starting position.

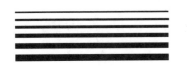

Combination Arm Reach

Cardiovascular Warm-Up

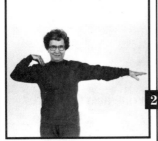

Start standing erect with hands on shoulders.

Straighten arm to one side.

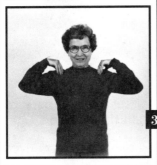

Return to starting position.

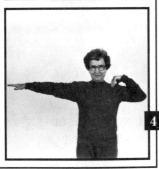

Straighten other arm to side.

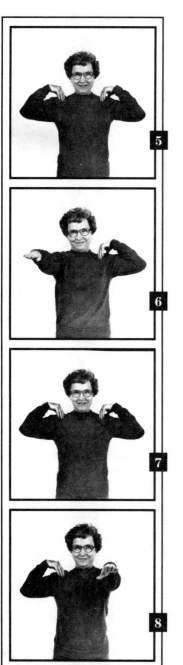

5 Return to starting position.

6 Straighten one arm forward.

7 Return to starting position.

8 Straighten other arm forward and return to starting position.

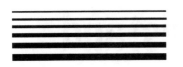

Arm Swings

Cardiovascular conditioning

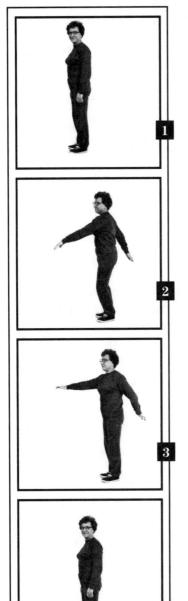

1 Start standing erect with arms at sides.

2 Swing one arm forward and other arm backward.

3 Swing arms in opposite directions, bending knees slightly on downswing.

4 Return to starting position.

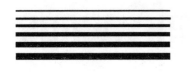

Twist and Clap

Cardiovascular conditioning

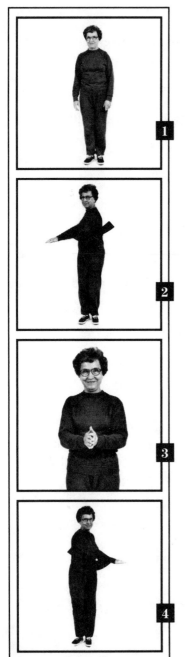

1 Start standing erect, feet slightly apart and arms at sides.

2 Twist upper body gently to side while bending knees slightly and swinging arms.

3 Return to center position and clap.

4 Twist body gently to other side, return to center, and clap.

Tip: Do not do this exercise if you have had back surgery.

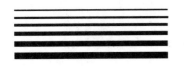

Toe Touch/ Foot Kick

Cardiovascular conditioning

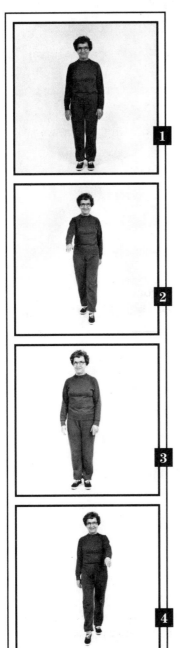

1 Start standing erect with feet slightly apart, arms at sides.

2 Touch one toe in front while swinging opposite arm forward.

3 Return to starting position.

4 Touch other toe in front while swinging opposite arm forward.

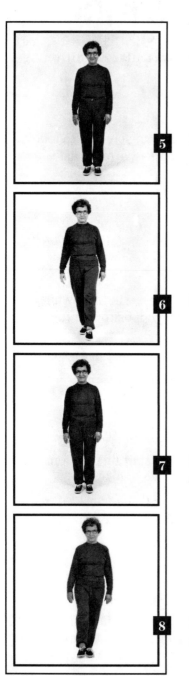

5 Return to starting position.

6 Kick one foot forward.

7 Return to starting position and repeat with other foot.

8 Kick other foot forward and return to starting position.

4

Exercise Routines

This chapter explains the routines used in the Over 50 and Fit program. These routines include various combinations of the exercises in Chapter Three.

First learn each exercise in a routine, giving yourself plenty of time to practice each exercise. Then combine the exercises, practicing your entire routine to music. Before long, you'll know all the exercise routines and spend your entire exercise sessions doing them to music!

During any one exercise session, be sure to include at least one warm-up routine, one aerobic routine, and one cool-down routine. Also monitor yourself regularly, using either the pulse method or the Exertion Scale.

Warm-Up Routine 1

Purpose: To start using all muscle groups; stretching muscles and preparing joints for safe activity.

Tip: Do warm-up exercises slowly and rhythmically with a natural flow from one to the next. Keep your breathing natural and regular and your body relaxed.

Standing

1. Neck Pendulum: two times

2. Head Turns: two times

3. Shoulder Circles: four times—both directions

4. Shoulder Shrugs: four times

5. Shoulder Arm Circles: four backward, four forward—alternating arms

6. Overhead Arm Reach: four times—each arm

7. Forward Reach: two times—each side

8. Side Stretch: two times—each side

9. Side Lunge: two times—each side

10. Calf Stretch: two times—each side

Warm-Up Routine 2

Purpose: To improve flexibility of lower back and legs.

Tip: Do stretches slowly without bouncing. Remember not to overdo it. Breathe in as you straighten up, and out as you lean forward.

Sitting on floor

1. Forward Stretch: two times

2. Straddle Stretch: two times—entire sequence

3. Flexed Straddle Stretch: two times

4. Combination Stretch: two times—each leg

Warm-Up Routine 3

Purpose: To strengthen and tone abdomen, lower back, and legs.

Tip: Keep your lower back rounded and not arched. Remember to exhale on exertion.

Sitting on floor; knees bent

1. Lower Leg Lift: three times—each leg

2. Total Leg Lift: two times—each leg

Lying on floor

3. Curl Down: two to four times

4. Curl Up (alternative Curl Down): two to four times

5. Knee Drop: two times—each leg

6. Leg Lowering I: two times—each leg, toe pointed

7. Leg Lowering II: two times—each leg, toe flexed

8. Side Leg Lift: four times—each leg

9. Pelvic Tilt: four times

Warm-Up Routine 4

Purpose: To provide overall strengthening and stretching.

Tip: Make sure not to hold your breath during exercises.

Sitting on chair

1. Lower Leg Lift: four times—each leg, each side

2. Forward Stretch: one time, hold

3. Crossed Ankle Lift: two times—each leg

4. Ankle Circles: four times—each leg, each direction

5. Body Twist: two times—each side, hold

6. Total Leg Lift: two times—each leg

7. Forward Stretch: one time, hold

Warm-Up Routine 5

Purpose: To stretch and strengthen lower body.

Tip: Make sure chairs are stable.

Standing behind chair

1. Heel Lift with Half Knee Bends: four to six times

2. Leg Swings: four times—each leg

3. Side Lunge: three times—each side

4. Calf Stretch: two times—each leg, each side

5. Repeat steps 1, 3, and 4

Cardiovascular Warm-Up Routine

Purpose: To gradually increase heart rate by increasing muscle work.

Tip: Watch out for overexertion.

1. Combination Arm Reach: four times—each arm, side and front

2. Arm Swings: eight swings—each arm

3. Twist and Clap: four times—each side

4. Toe Touch/Foot Kick: eight times—each side

5. Walking to music

Aerobic Routine 1

Purpose: To gradually raise and maintain heart rate in Target Zone for five to ten minutes by exercising muscle groups rhythmically and continuously.

Tip: Watch for signs of overexertion (heavy breathing, leg or arm fatigue, or dizziness). To increase your heart rate, lift your knees higher. If you tend to get dizzy walking backward, simply turn and walk forward.

1. March forward seven steps; clap
   March backward seven steps; clap

Repeat

2. Step to the right three steps; clap hands above head
   Step to the left three steps; clap hands by knees

Repeat

3. March forward seven steps; clap
   March backward seven steps; clap

4. March in place eight steps
   Repeat entire sequence one to four times

Aerobic Routine 2

Purpose: To gradually raise and maintain heart rate in Target Zone for five to ten minutes by exercising muscle groups rhythmically and continuously.

Tip: If you begin to get too tired, then omit arm movements, slow down the walk, or do both.

Walk throughout this routine

1. Walk to the right 16 steps, then to the left 16 steps

2. Single Arm Reaches (continue walking to left)
   Side—four times with each arm
   Front—four times with each arm
   Down—four times with each arm

3. Walk to the right 16 steps, then to the left 16 steps

4. Arm Reaches—both arms in unison
   (continue walking to left)
   Side—four times
   Front—four times
   Side—four times
   Front—four times

5. Walk to the right 16 steps, then to the left 16 steps

6. Walk in place

Aerobic Routine 3

Purpose: To gradually raise and maintain heart rate in Target Zone for five to ten minutes by exercising muscle groups rhythmically and continuously.

Tip: If you are not able to raise and maintain your heart rate in your Target Zone, do steps 1 and 2 in double-time or add arm swings.

1. Walk forward eight steps
   Walk backward eight steps

Repeat

2. Up on toes with arms stretched overhead—walk forward eight steps
   Hands on knees—walk backward eight steps

3. Walk forward eight steps
   Walk backward eight steps

4. Walk in place four steps

5. Walk forward with eight step-knee lifts
   Turn to right side—walk backward with eight sidesteps
   Repeat turning to the left side while walking backward
   Repeat entire sequence, steps 1 through 5

Cool-Down Routine 1

Purpose: To lower heart rate by reducing activity.

Tip: Remember to relax through the entire routine, breathing deeply.

Walking slowly throughout

1. Shoulder Shrugs: four times

2. Elbow Circles/Elbow Press: circle three times—both directions, press together

3. Overhead Arm Reach: two times—each arm

4. Walks: Toe, Heel, Duck, Pigeon: eight steps—each position

5. Repeat steps 1 through 4

Cool-Down Routine 2

Purpose: To relax muscles and bring heart rate close to normal.

Tip: Make sure to relax through entire routine, breathing deeply.

Sitting on chair or standing

1. Wrist Circles: four times—each direction

2. Palm Rotation: four times

3. Finger Flex: two times—each finger

4. Neck Pendulum: two times

5. Repeat steps 1 through 4

5

Alternative Exercises

The exercises included in this chapter provide just some of the many ways you can add variety and increase the level of exertion in your workouts. In addition, you'll find two additional aerobic routines, exercises for people with arthritis, and a breathing exercise. Just remember that a balanced exercise session includes a warm-up period, an aerobic workout, and a cool-down period.

Other activities that will provide you with the benefits of aerobic exercise include dancing, swimming, skiing, bicycling, hiking, and cross-country skiing.

With various kinds of exercise equipment, you can also get a good aerobic workout without leaving your house. One popular example is the stationary bicycle. Another is the jogging trampoline, which allows you to get the benefits of jogging with less stress on your joints. However, you might experience loss of balance and dizziness while jumping on a trampoline. Be cautious if you use one, or use a model that has a support bar.

Variety is a key element in a successful exercise program. New additions to your regular routine will help keep you motivated to continue exercising. Challenge yourself with new, if not more advanced exercises from examples in this chapter.

The following alternative exercises can easily be done with household objects—for example, vegetable cans, books, or lightweight dumbbells (under five pounds). Start by using a weight that challenges you without overexerting you. Remember to be patient with yourself and to focus on your individual progress.

Start all exercises with four repetitions and work up to ten.

Single Arm Reaches

Strengthens shoulders and upper back

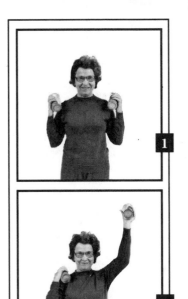

Start standing or sitting, holding objects at shoulder level with overhand grip.

Extend one arm overhead; lower. Repeat with other arm.

Tip: Remember to breathe normally throughout the exercise. Exhale on exertion, inhale on relaxation.

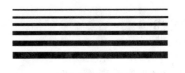

Arm Curls

Strengthens upper arms

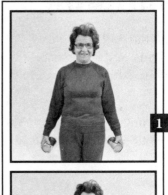

1

Start standing or sitting, holding objects with underhand grips at sides.

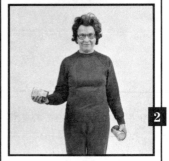

2

Bend elbow, raising object until arm is fully bent; lower. Repeat with other arm.

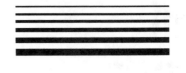

Arm Extension

**Strengthens back of
upper arms and increases
range of motion**

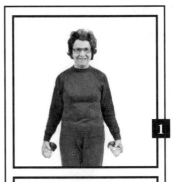

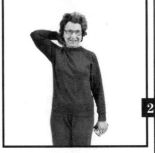

Start standing or sitting, holding
objects with underhand grips at
sides.

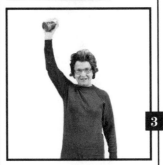

Extend one arm overhead, holding object. Lower object behind
back, as far as comfortable.

Return same arm overhead and
lower to side. Repeat with other
arm.

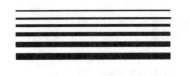

Half Squats

Strengthens thigh muscles

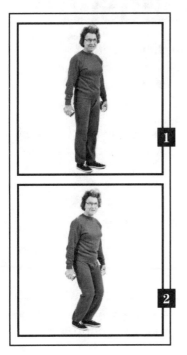

1 Start by holding object in each hand, arms at sides.

2 Slowly bend knees to a 45-degree angle; return to upright position.

Arm Press

Strengthens chest muscles

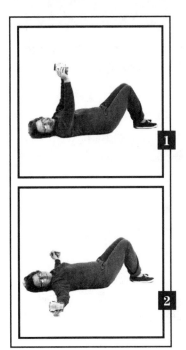

Start by lying on back with knees bent; grasp object in each hand and extend arms over chest.

Lower arms out to sides with arms slightly bent.

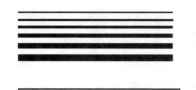

Backswing Extension

Strengthens chest, arm, and shoulder muscles

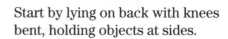

Start by lying on back with knees bent, holding objects at sides.

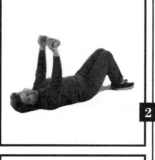

Slowly lift objects over chest with straight arms.

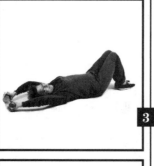

Lower straight arms back to floor.

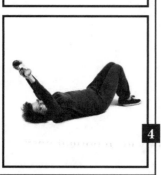

Swing arms upward over chest and down to starting position.

Tip: Do not arch back; keep middle of back on floor.

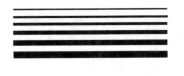

Advanced Curl Ups

Strengthens abdominal muscles

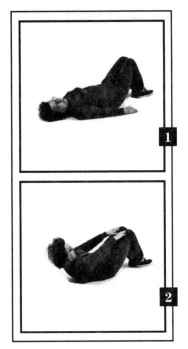

1 Start lying on back with knees bent and arms at sides.

2 Raise up to a 45-degree angle reaching forward with arms.

Tip: Folding arms across chest increases the workload.

Advanced Side Leg Lift

Strengthens outside thigh muscle

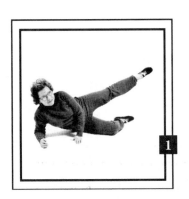

1 Start by lying on side, supporting your body in an upright position. Raise upper leg to a 45-degree angle, then lower.

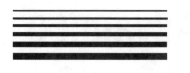

Advanced Stretching

Intensifies muscle stretch and increases range of motion in the joints

You will need a 24-inch-long broomstick or twisted towel to do this group of broomstick exercises. You can do them while standing or sitting.

Broomstick Twist

Stretches upper back and midriff

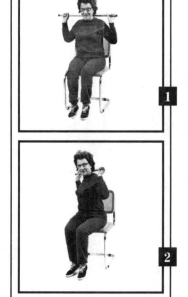

1 Start by sitting in chair, holding broomstick behind neck, elbows bent.

2 Twist shoulders and upper body to the right and to the left.

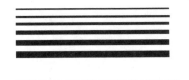

Broomstick Lift and Lower

**Stretches shoulders
and upper back**

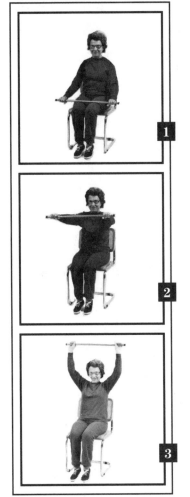

1 Start by sitting in chair, holding broomstick or towel with hands approximately 24 inches apart on knees.

2 Lift broomstick to shoulder level.

3 Lift broomstick over head.

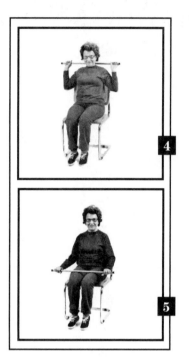

4 Lower broomstick behind neck to shoulder level.

5 Lift broomstick up, bring forward and down to knees.

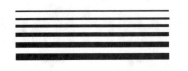

Broomstick Side Stretch

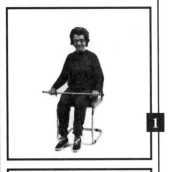

1 Start by sitting in a chair, holding broomstick on knees.

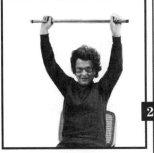

2 Lift broomstick over head with arms extended.

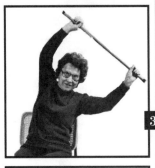

3 Stretch arms and shoulders to one side.

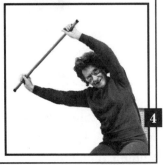

4 Stretch arms and shoulders to the other side.

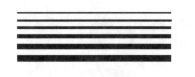

Forward Reach and Floor Touch

Stretches upper and lower back

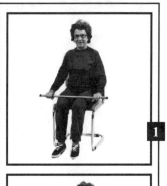

1 Start by standing or sitting in a chair, holding broomstick on knees.

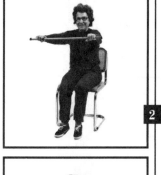

2 Push broomstick away from you at chest level.

3 Extend broomstick and reach forward as far as possible.

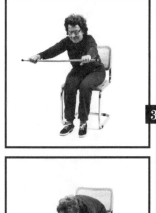

4 Curl forward and touch toes with broomstick; return to starting position.

Tip: If standing, omit step 4.

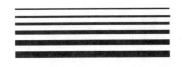

Wrist Flex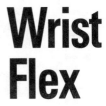

Increases wrist flexibility

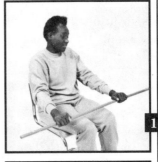

Start by sitting in a chair, holding broomstick with overhand grip.

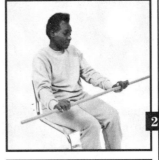

Flex wrists up, bringing hands toward chest.

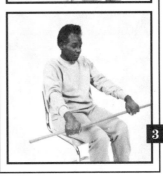

Flex wrists down, bringing hands toward legs.

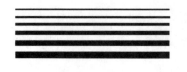

Criss-Cross

**Stretches shoulders
and upper back**

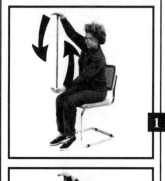

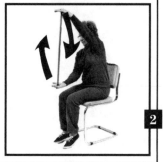

1 Start by sitting in a chair holding
the broomstick ends between the
palms of your hands, with the
right hand on top; arms straight.

2 Turn the stick, bringing the left
arm on the top; return to starting
position.

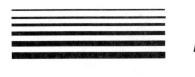

Alternative Aerobics

Aerobic Routine 4

Purpose: To gradually raise and maintain heart rate in Target Zone for five to ten minutes by exercising muscle groups rhythmically and continuously.

Tips: Lift knees higher to increase heart rate. If you are tired, slow your pace.

1. March 16 steps in place
   March 16 steps making a circle

2. March three steps to the right; kick
   March three steps to the left; kick

Repeat

3. March three steps forward; kick
   March three steps backward; kick

Repeat

4. Repeat steps 2 and 3, clapping hands as you kick

5. Relax eight beats

Repeat entire sequence

Aerobic Routine 5

Note: This routine calls for exercising with a partner.

Tip: If you feel tired, omit hops during the schottische pattern.

STARTING POSITION: Stand with a partner holding hands. Begin heel-toe swing pattern with the right foot, then with the left.

1. Heel-toe swing pattern; four heel-toe swings

   Do heel-toe swing pattern four times

2. Schottische pattern:
   three steps, one hop
   three steps, one hop
   four step-hops

   Do schottische pattern four times

3. Repeat steps 1 and 2

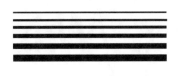

Arthritis and Fitness

Arthritis is a condition that requires special attention in an exercise program. Painful joints make it difficult for people with arthritis to exercise at times, yet exercise is crucial to maintaining joint movement.

Consistent stretching exercises help prevent deformity in the joints and enable you to continue performing daily tasks. The following exercises give additional resources for maintaining joint mobility.

If you have arthritis, keep these tips in mind:

1. Do all of the exercises slowly. Hold positions eight to ten seconds.

2. Start with three repetitions of each exercise and work up to ten.

3. Exercise every other day.

4. Warm up muscles by walking for a few minutes prior to stretching exercises.

5. You may feel some discomfort during the exercises. Try to stay below the pain level.

6. When joints are acutely inflamed and painful, keep movement to a minimum, or possibly supported in proper alignment, until sharp pain decreases.

7. If joints are painful after exercise, apply ice packs.

8. If your arthritis flares up severely on the day after exercise, it's a sign that you overdid exercising. Reduce your pace the next time you exercise.

Finger/Wrist Stretch

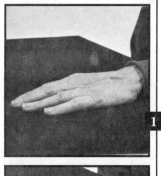

Start by sitting with arm resting on table, palm down.

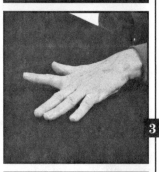

Spread fingers apart and bring them back together.

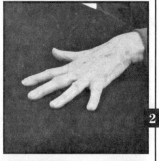

Lift each finger individually, keeping palm pressed against table.

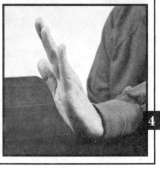

Lift entire hand off table, bending the wrist as far back as possible; repeat with other hand.

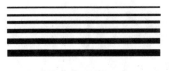

Wrist Switch

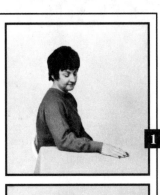

1 Start by sitting with arm resting on table, elbow bent to 90-degree angle, palm down.

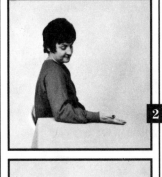

2 Turn hand so palm faces up and return to starting position.

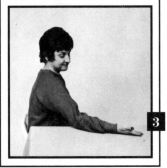

3 Straighten elbow, turn palm up and down. Repeat sequence with other hand.

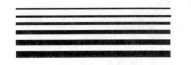

Wrist Switch with Hammer

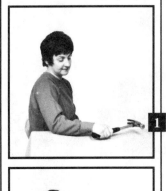

Start by sitting with arm resting on table or arm of chair, elbow bent to a 90-degree angle, grasping light hammer, palm down.

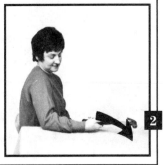

Turn hand so palm faces up. Repeat with other hand.

Hammer Circles

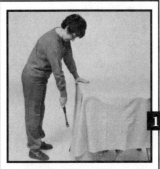

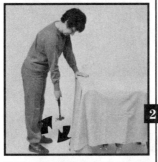

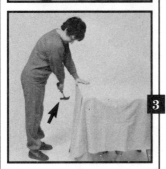

Start by leaning forward with one arm resting on table or armchair in front of you, holding light hammer down to one side with other arm. Relax and feel weight of arm.

Begin making small circles, keeping arm straight.

Swing arm across front of body and back and forth along side of body. Repeat with other arm.

Tip: Do not twist wrist. Motion should come from shoulders.

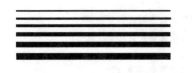

Angel Stretch

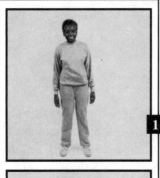

1 Start by standing or lying on back, arms at sides.

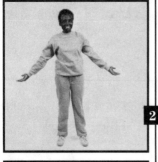

2 Lift arms up and out to sides, keeping elbows straight.

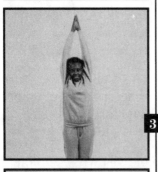

3 Continue movement; touch hands over head if possible.

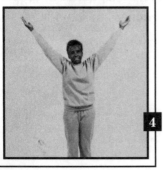

4 Swing arms back down.

Heel-Toe Rock

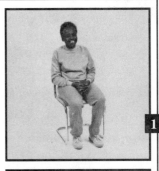

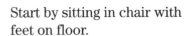 Start by sitting in chair with feet on floor.

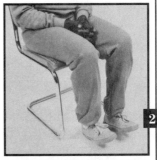

2 Lift toes off floor, keeping heels on floor. Return to feet flat on floor.

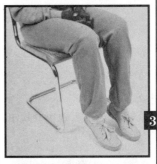

3 Lift heels off floor, keeping toes on floor. Return to feet flat on floor.

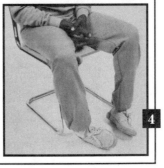

4 Roll each foot out to the side by lifting inside of the foot. Return to feet flat on floor.

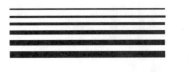

Knee Tuck

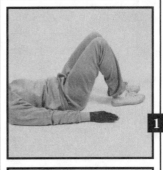

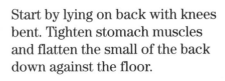

Start by lying on back with knees bent. Tighten stomach muscles and flatten the small of the back down against the floor.

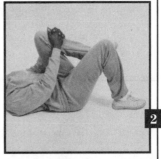

Bring one knee up toward chest. Grasp knee with hands and pull toward chest until you feel a good stretch (but not pain) in the back muscles.

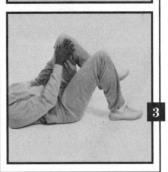

Slowly lower the leg back to starting position. Repeat, using the other knee.

Tip: Keep back pressed against the floor.

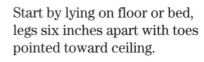

Leg Stretch

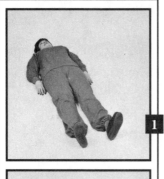

Start by lying on floor or bed, legs six inches apart with toes pointed toward ceiling.

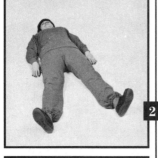

Move one leg out to the side and return. Move other leg out to the side and return.

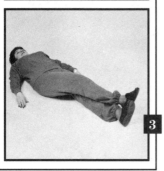

Cross one leg over the other leg and return. Repeat with other leg.

Tip: To increase resistance on the muscles, use an exercise belt or piece of elastic around your ankles.

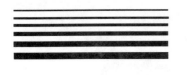

Breathing Exercise

Breathing in the proper sequence is a good way to exercise the major respiratory muscles. These muscles need proper exercise to remain strong and efficient.

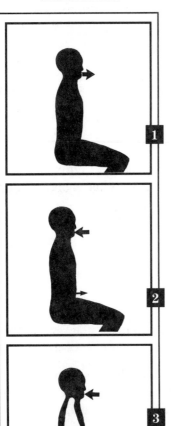

1 Start by sitting up straight in a chair and exhaling completely.

2 Inhale slowly and deeply, through your nose, keeping your stomach muscles relaxed.

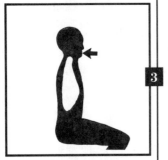

3 Fill your chest with air, expanding your lower ribs. Take at least five seconds to do this.

Tip: While inhaling, place your hand on your stomach. If you feel your stomach rise as your lungs fill with air, you are breathing properly.

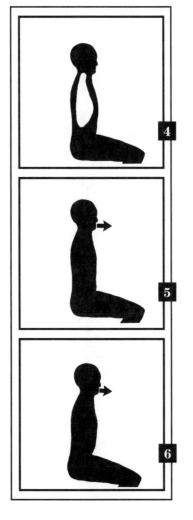

4 Hold for a few seconds.

5 Exhale gradually, controlling the release of air while relaxing your chest and rib cage.

6 Slowly pull in your abdominal muscles, forcing the remaining air out. DO NOT SLUMP FORWARD.

Practice this method of breathing once or twice a day. As you become more familiar with the exercise, you will be able to slow down your rate of breathing and increase your repetitions.

The benefits of regular breathing exercises are many. Your respiratory system will become more efficient, and you will feel calm, refreshed, and relaxed.

Glossary

Aerobic—Oxygen-using; describes heart-lung or stamina exercise. Aerobic exercise is steady, "nonstop" activity. Examples include calisthenics, swimming, jogging, and walking.

Anaerobic—Exercise that is short in duration, "stop and go" in rhythm, and low intensity in effort. Examples include tennis and golf.

Cardio—Pertaining to the heart.

Calisthenics—Systematic, rhythmic exercise.

Endurance—Ability to exercise continuously for a period of time.

Flexibility—Ability to move limbs through a range of joint motions.

Hypertension—High blood pressure.

Hyperextension—An extreme or abnormal stretch of a joint.

Isometric—Muscle contraction without movement; static exercise.

Isotonic—Muscle contraction with movement; rhythmic, repetitive exercise.

Pulmonary—Pertaining to the lungs.

Pulse—Regular beat felt in the arteries caused by contractions of the heart muscle.

Target Heart Rate Zone—A safe pulse range for exercising, adjusted for age.

Vascular—Pertaining to blood vessels, arteries, and veins.

Vein—Tube-like vessel that carries deoxygenated blood to the heart.